AF594780

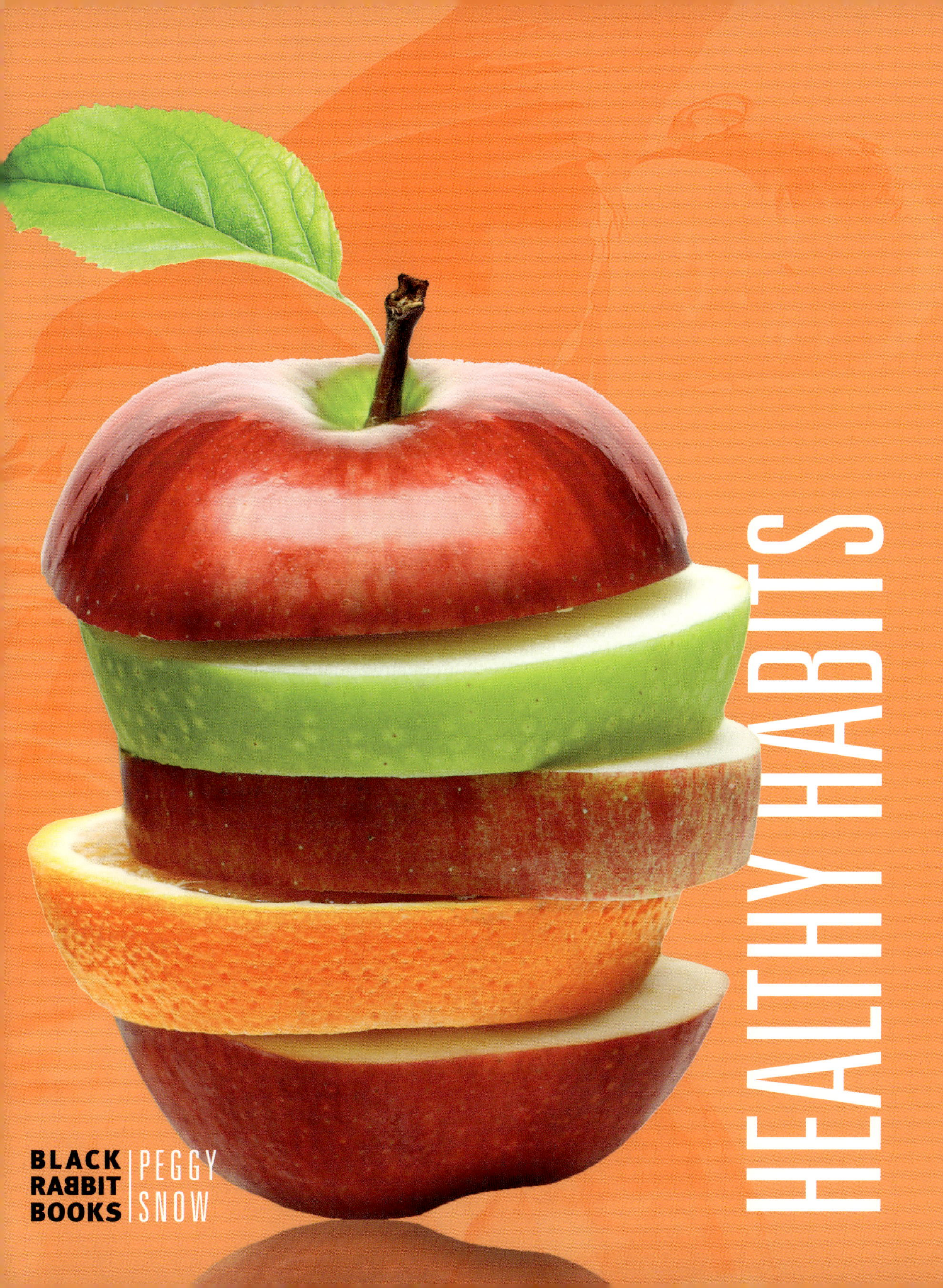

HEALTHY HABITS
BLACK RABBIT BOOKS
PEGGY SNOW

TABLE OF CONTENTS

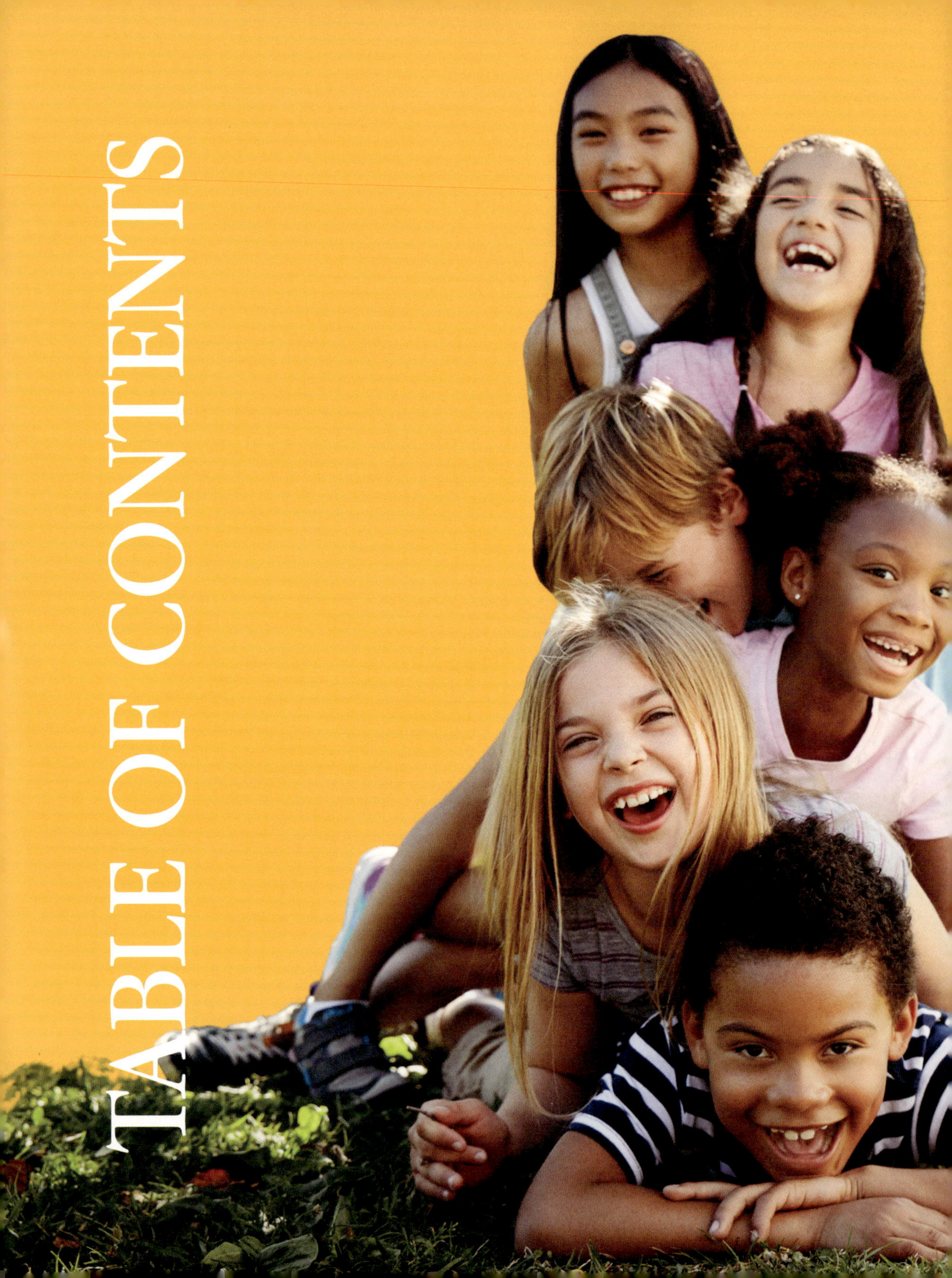

1. Play and Have Fun 4

2. Hang Out with Friends 6

3. Eat Right 10

4. Relax 13

5. Keep Your Body Clean 16

6. Get Enough Sleep 19

More to Explore 22

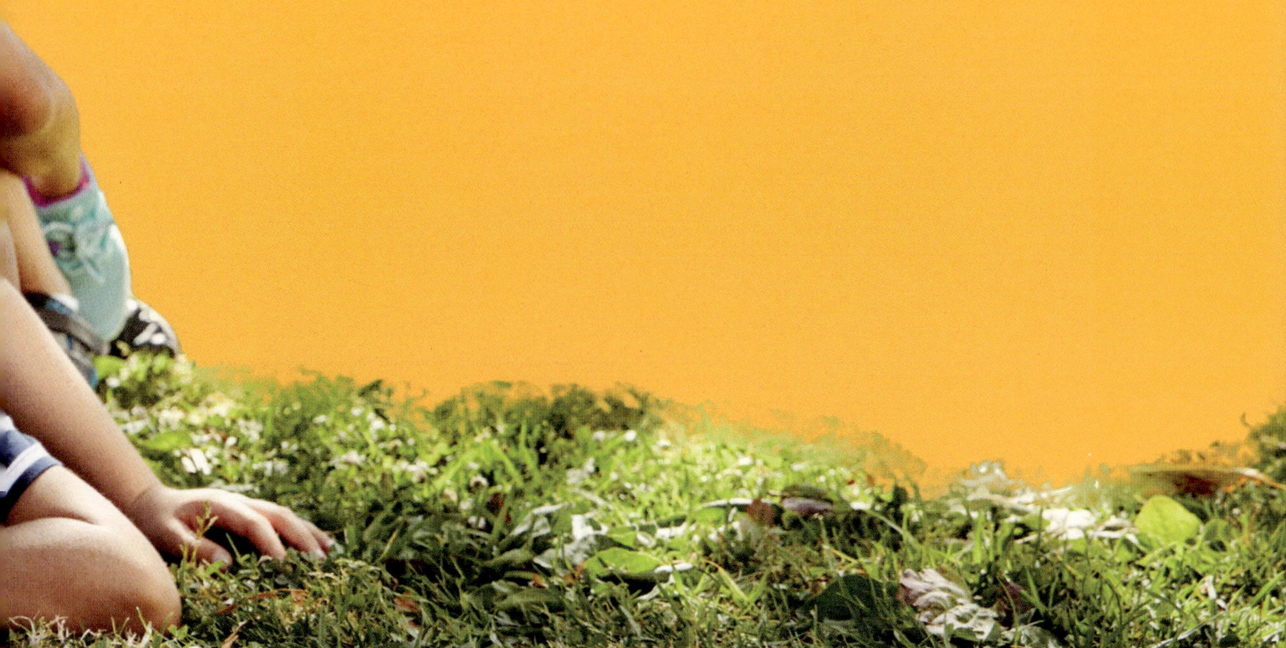

1

Play and Have Fun

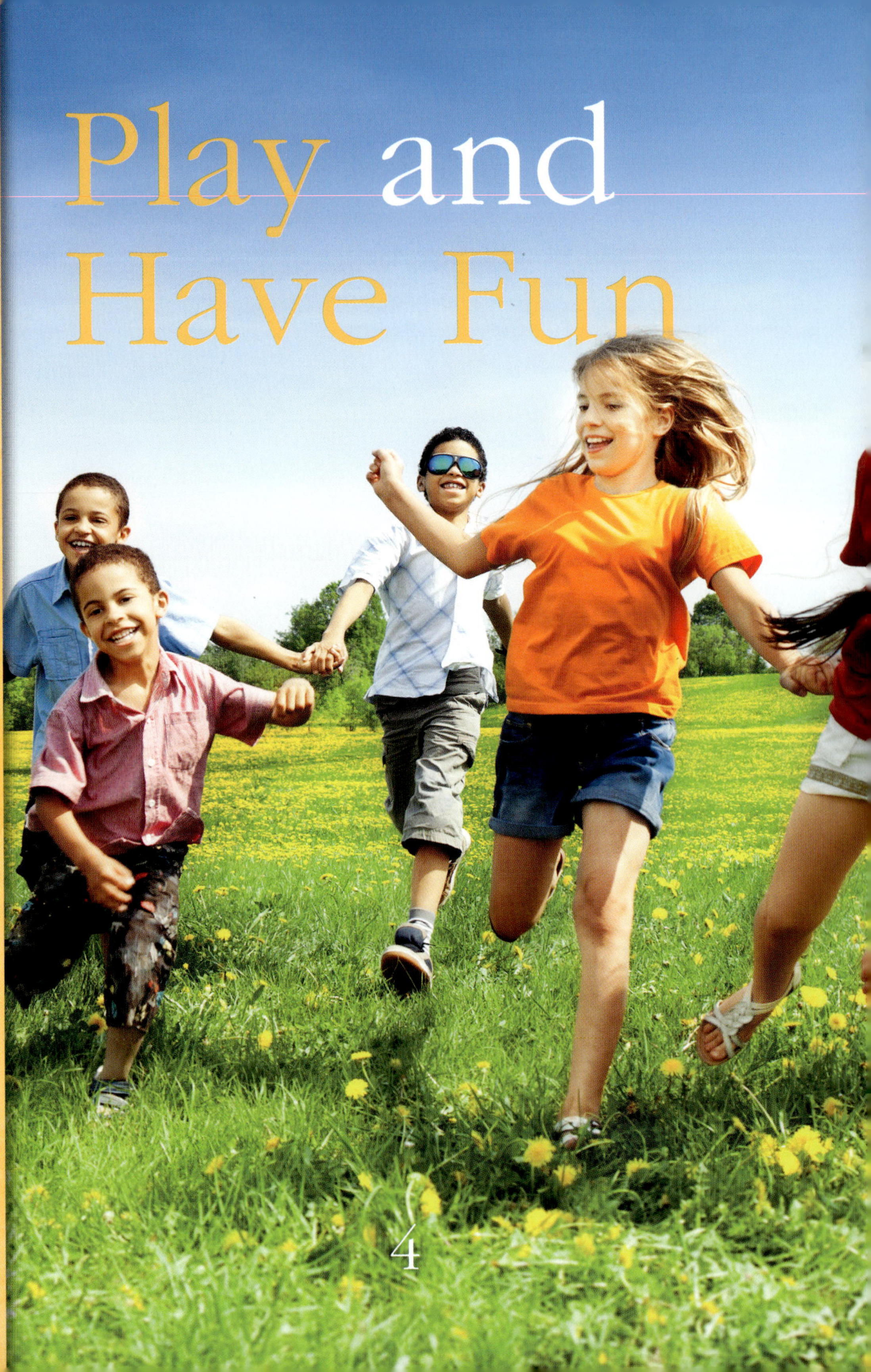

Habits are things you do often. It is important to build good habits. These will keep you healthy.

Having fun is healthy for your body and mind. When you play soccer or run on the playground, you strengthen your heart and lungs. You build muscles and strong bones. Your brain releases feel-good chemicals. This puts you in a better mood. Being happy is healthy.

Playing board games develops your brain. When you play Yahtzee, you learn math. Games like Connect 4 help you learn strategy.

Think About It

Your body needs one hour of physical activity each day. How do you get active?

2

Hang Out with Friends

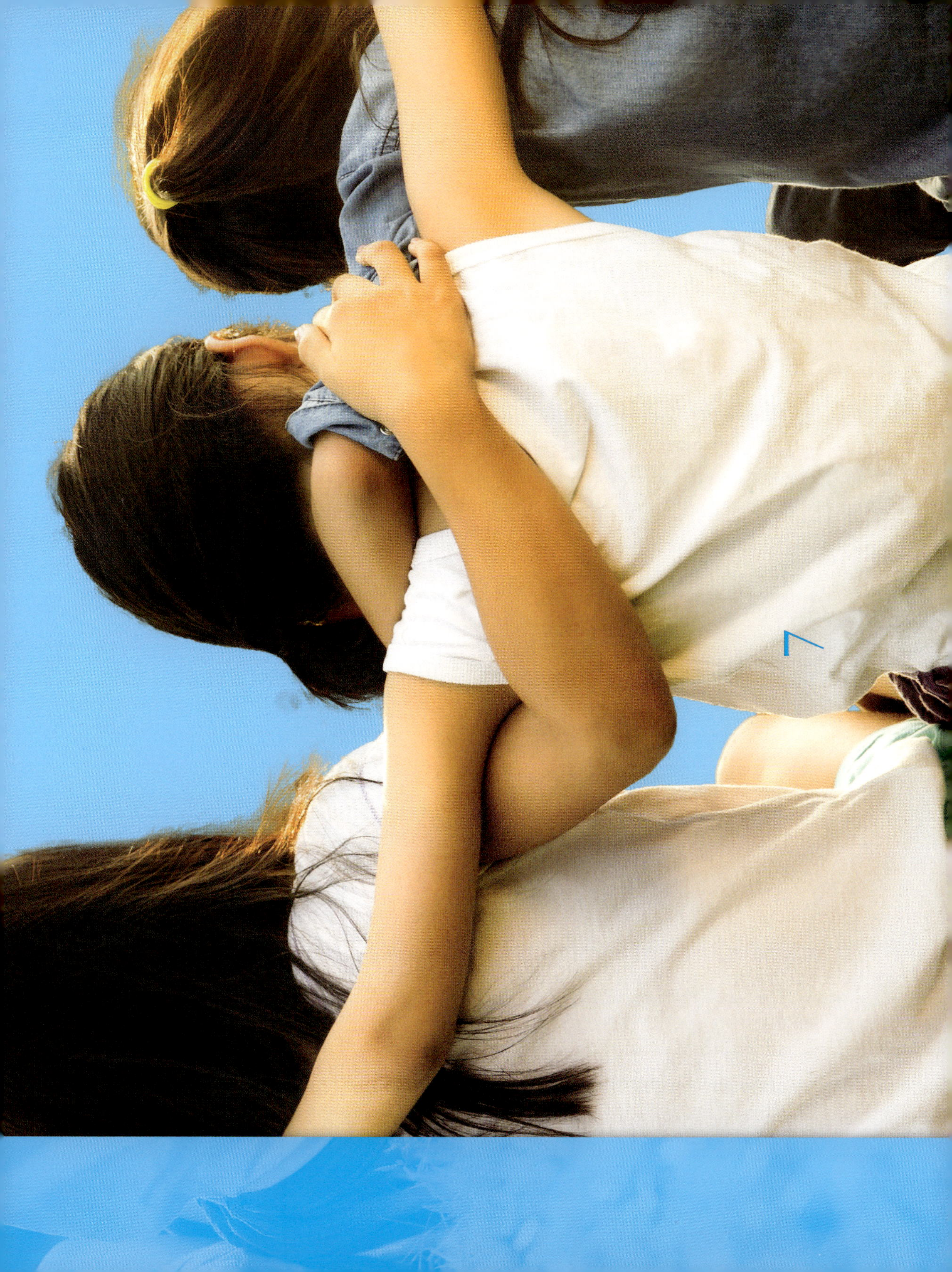

Being around people you like is good for your health. Spending time with friends builds your self-esteem.

Feeling good about yourself is healthy for your body. It helps your immune system.

Hanging out with friends can lift your mood. This happens when you play games, listen to music, or do homework together.

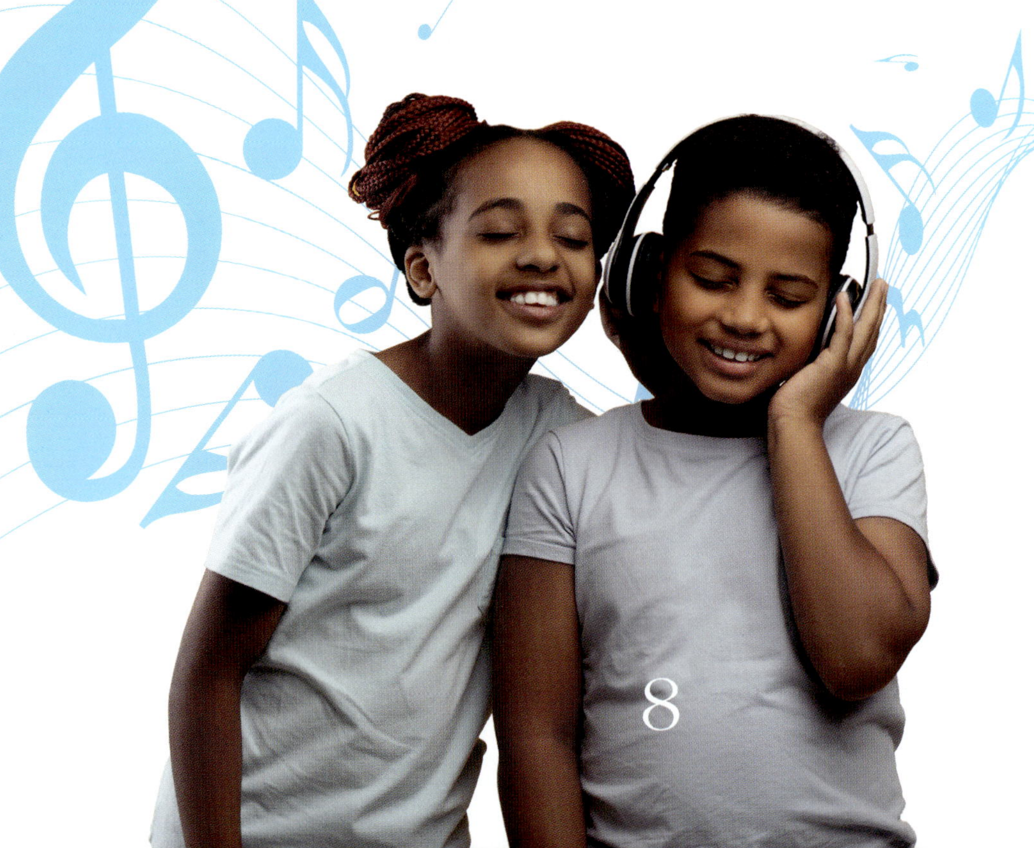

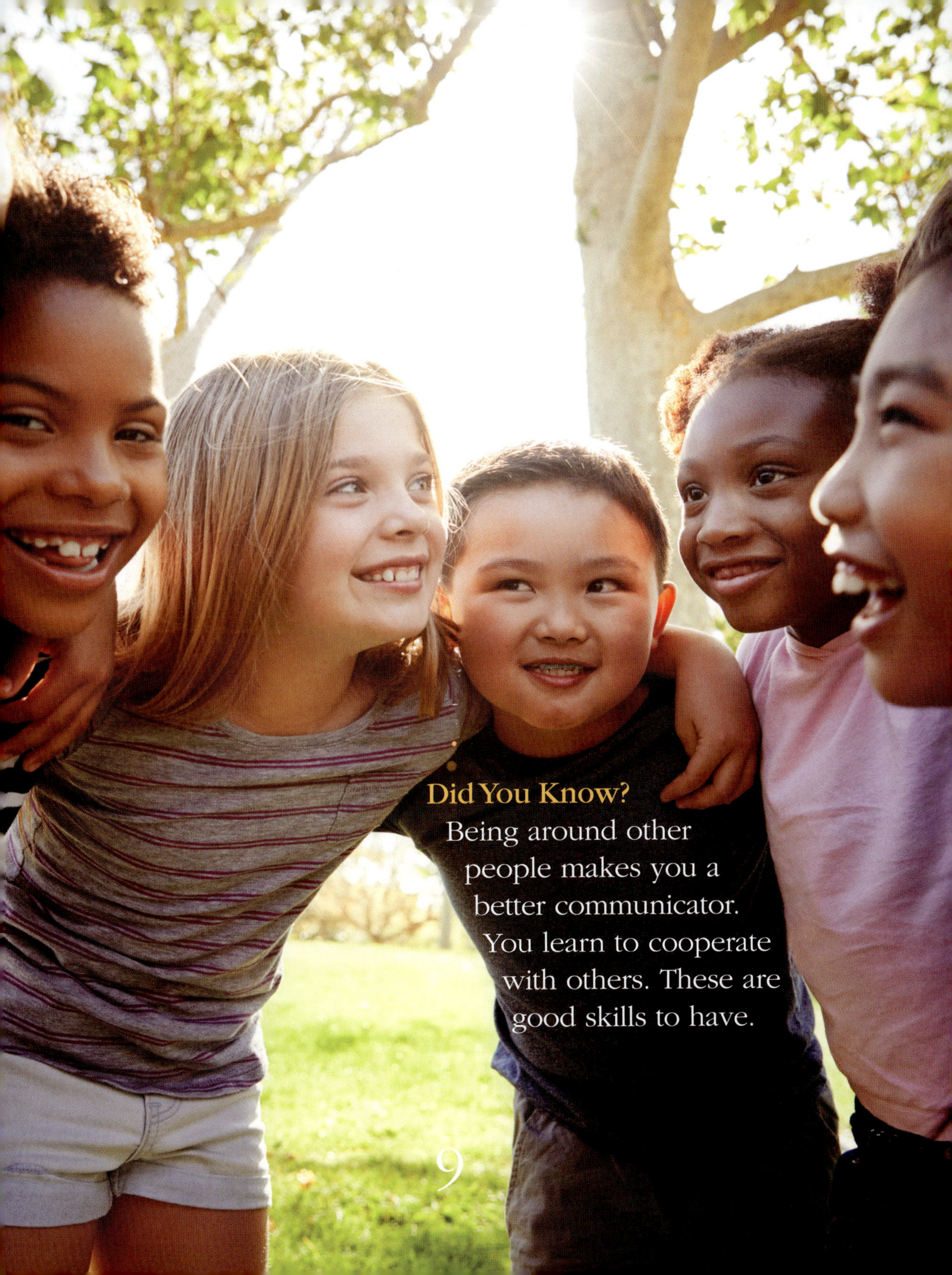

Did You Know?

Being around other people makes you a better communicator. You learn to cooperate with others. These are good skills to have.

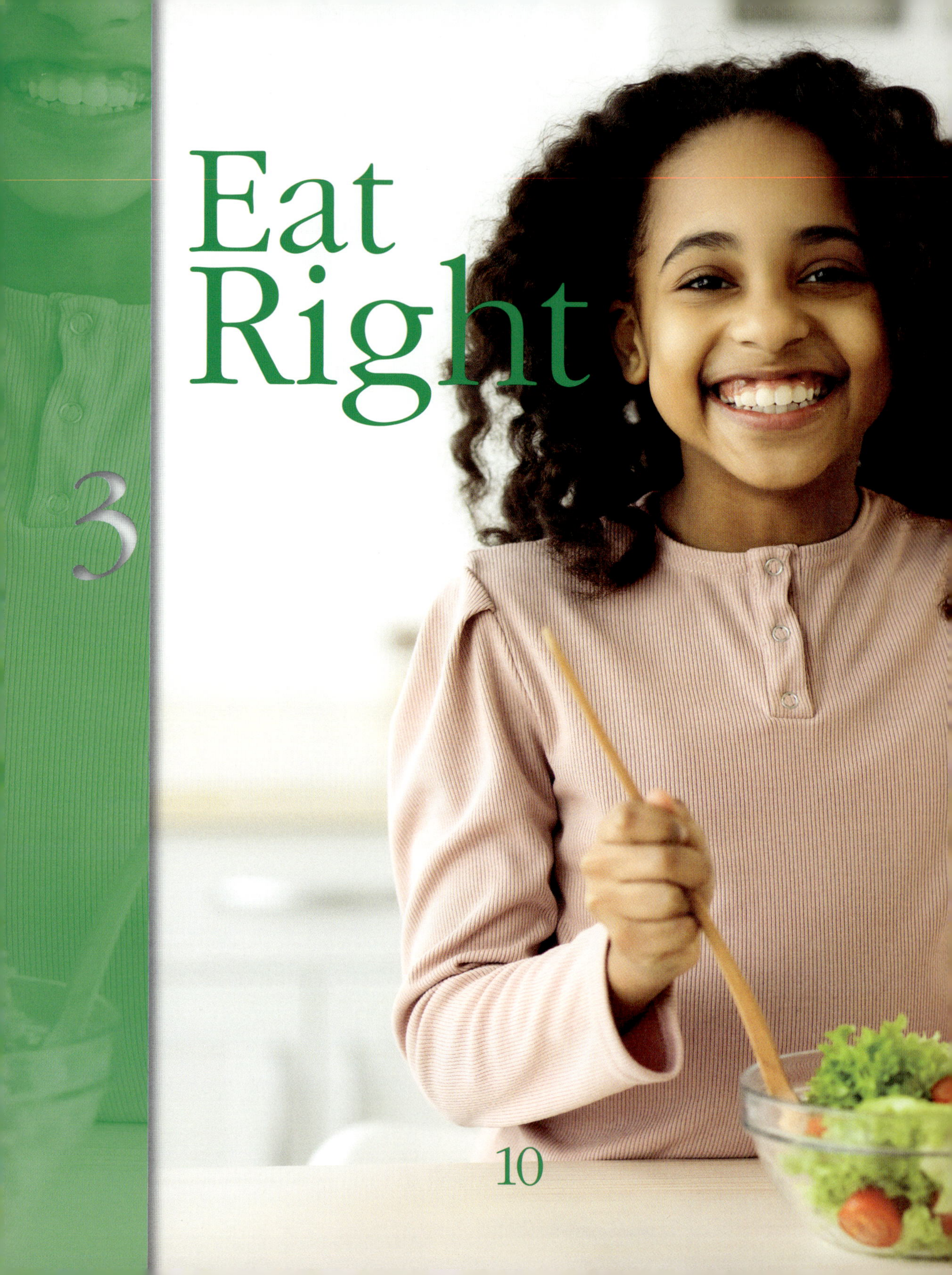

3

Eat Right

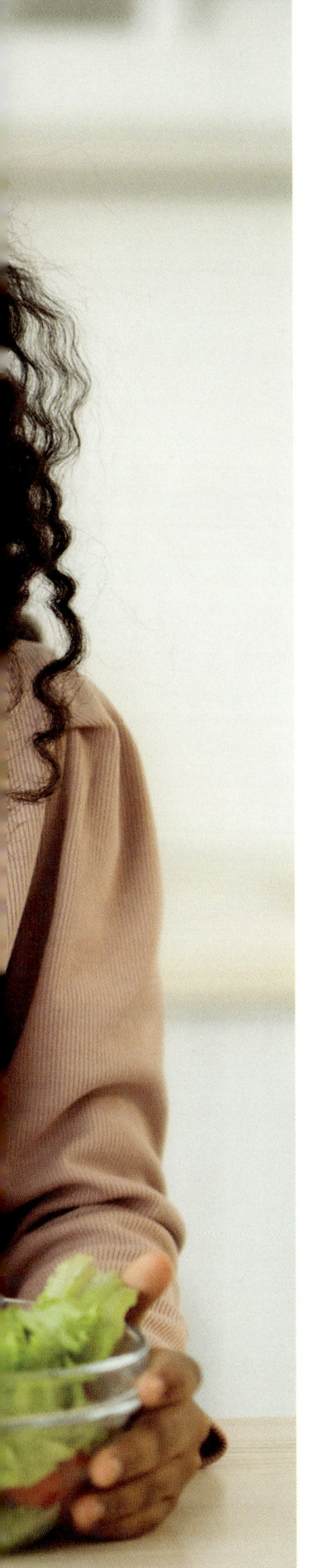

Healthy foods supply the nutrients your body needs. This helps you grow. And it gives you energy to play and have fun.

A good habit is to eat colorful food. Red tomatoes, blueberries, yellow bananas, and green veggies are full of vitamins and minerals.

Try to eat a vegetable or some fruit with every meal. Apples, raisins, and carrots are good choices for snacks.

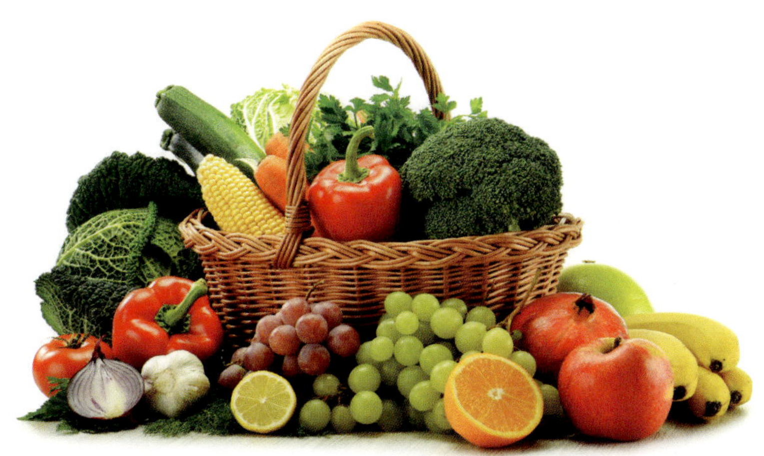

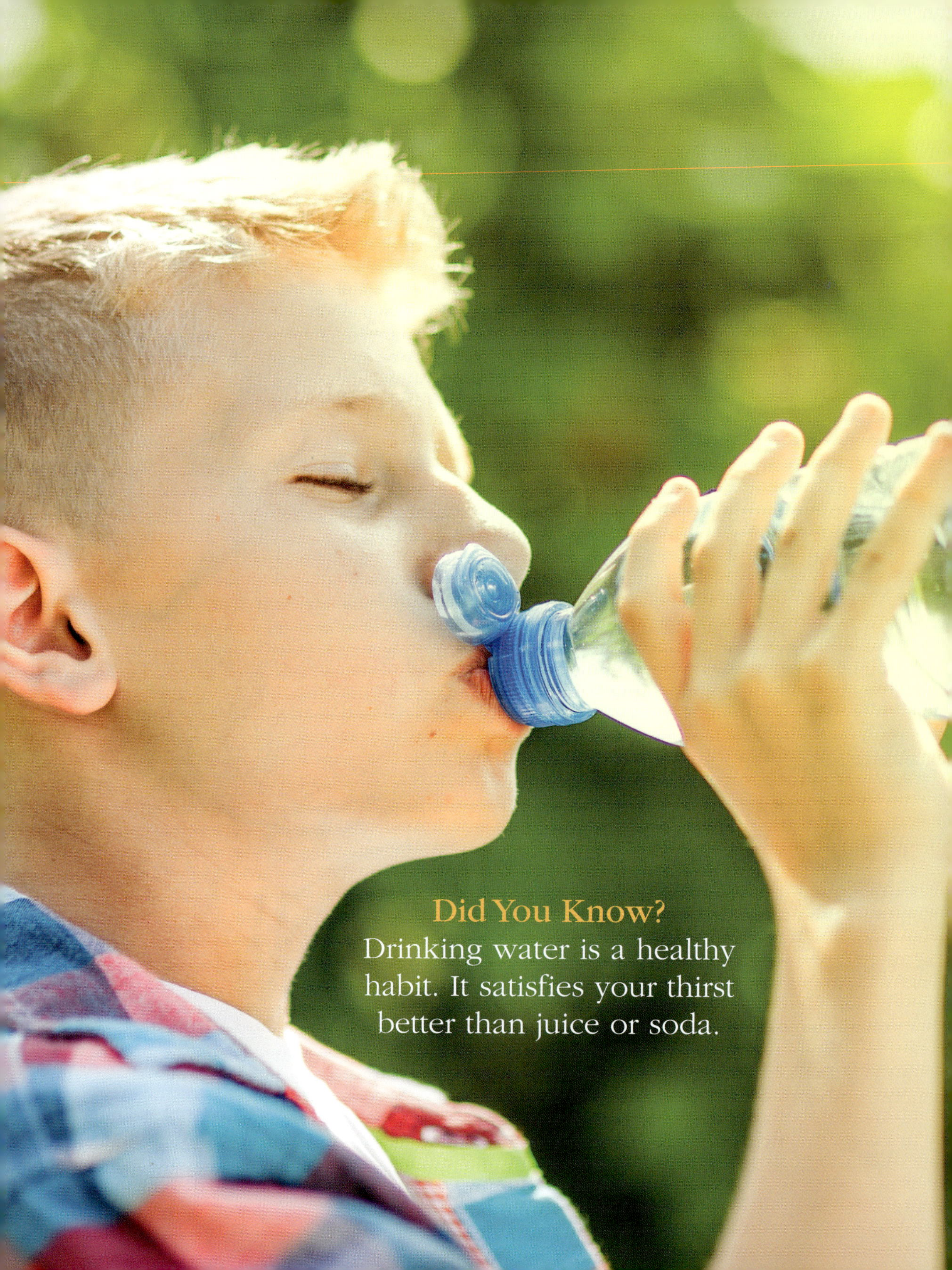

Did You Know?
Drinking water is a healthy habit. It satisfies your thirst better than juice or soda.

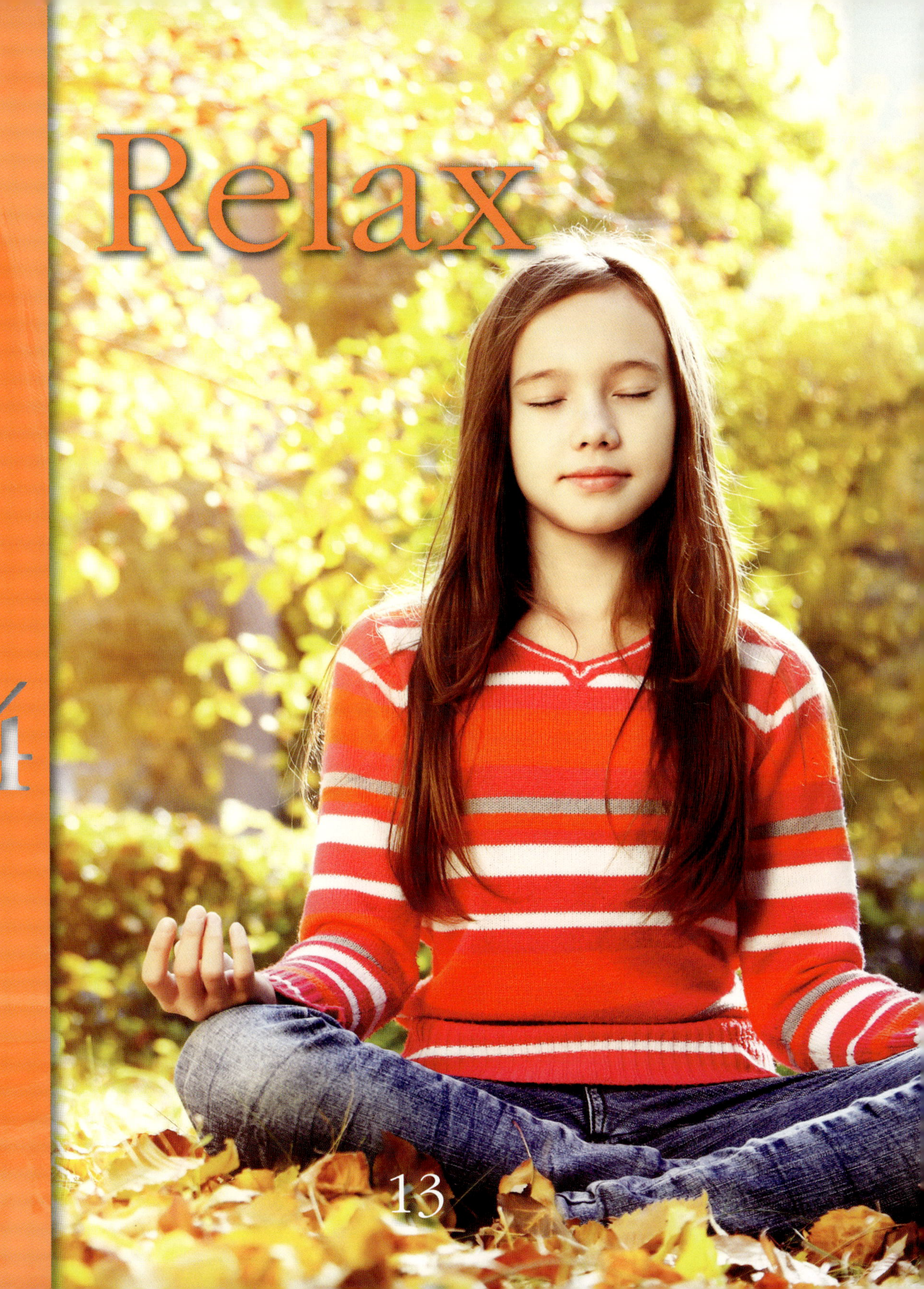

4

Relax

Take time to relax every day. Spend 10 to 15 minutes unwinding. Read, draw, or daydream. Try **meditation** or deep breathing. Or just sit quietly with your eyes closed.

If your body feels tight or tired, stretch or do yoga. Take a nap if you can. Naps aren't just for babies and old people. They can help you feel more **alert**.

Relaxing calms your mind. It relieves stress and **tension**. It helps you sleep better at night.

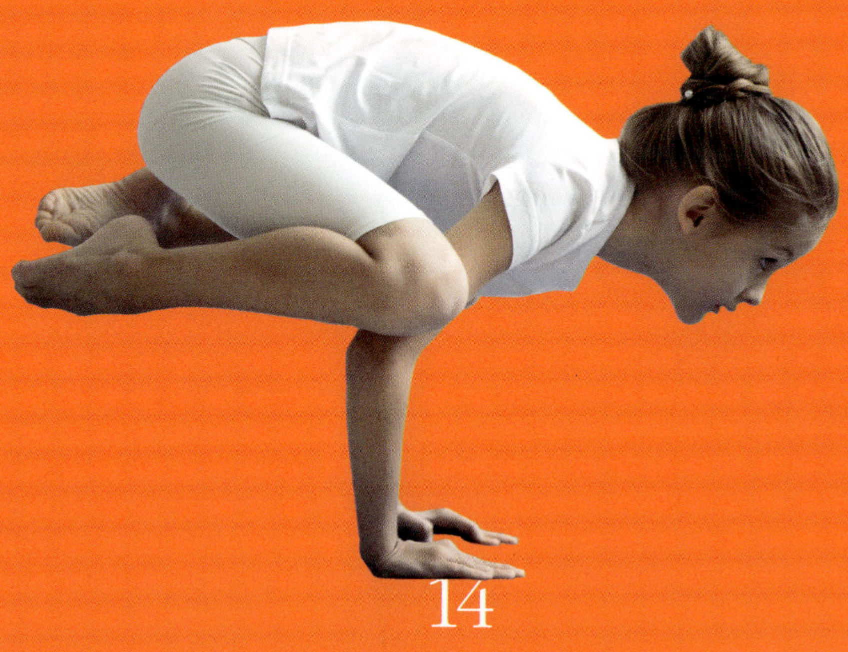

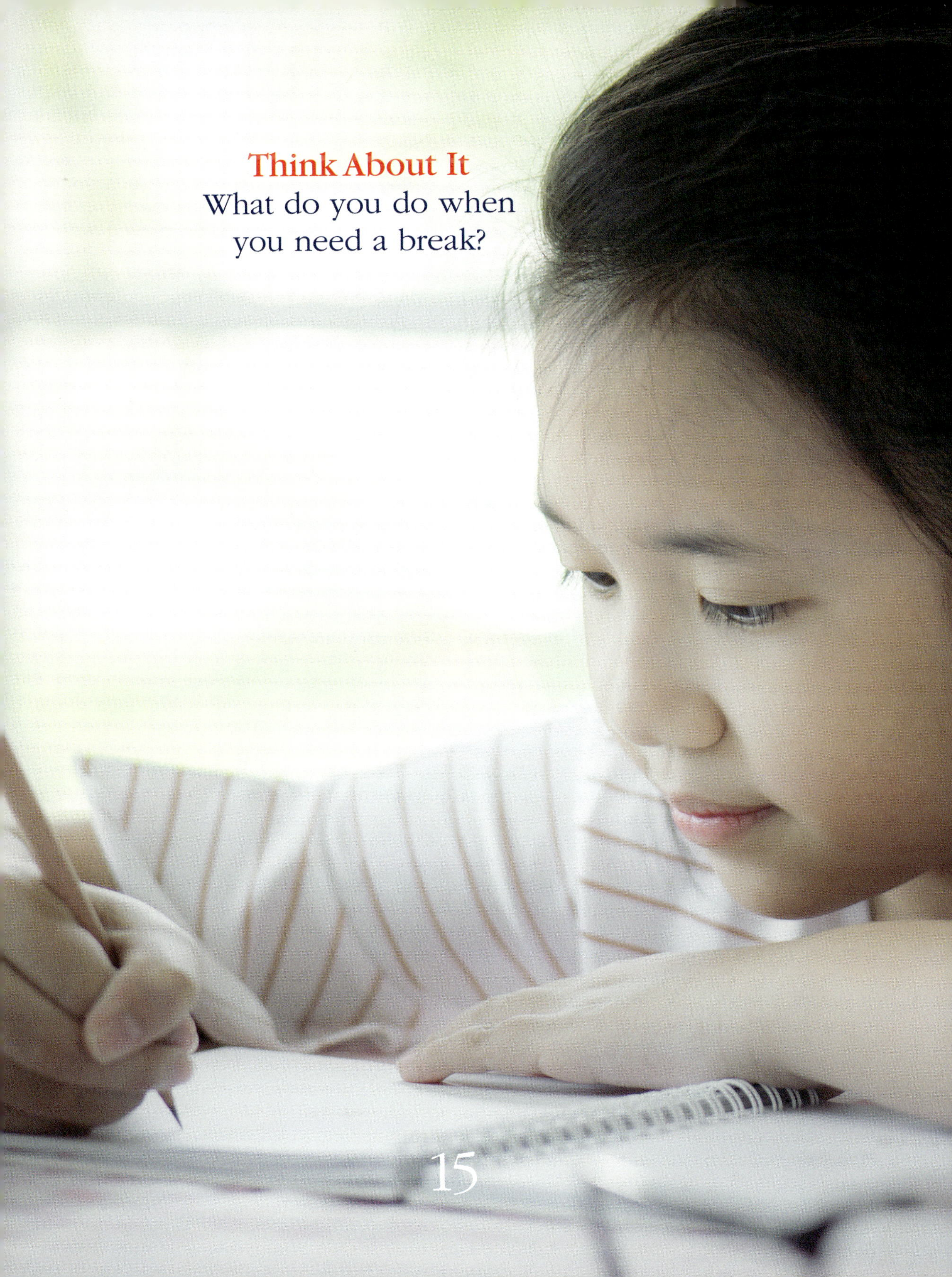

Think About It

What do you do when you need a break?

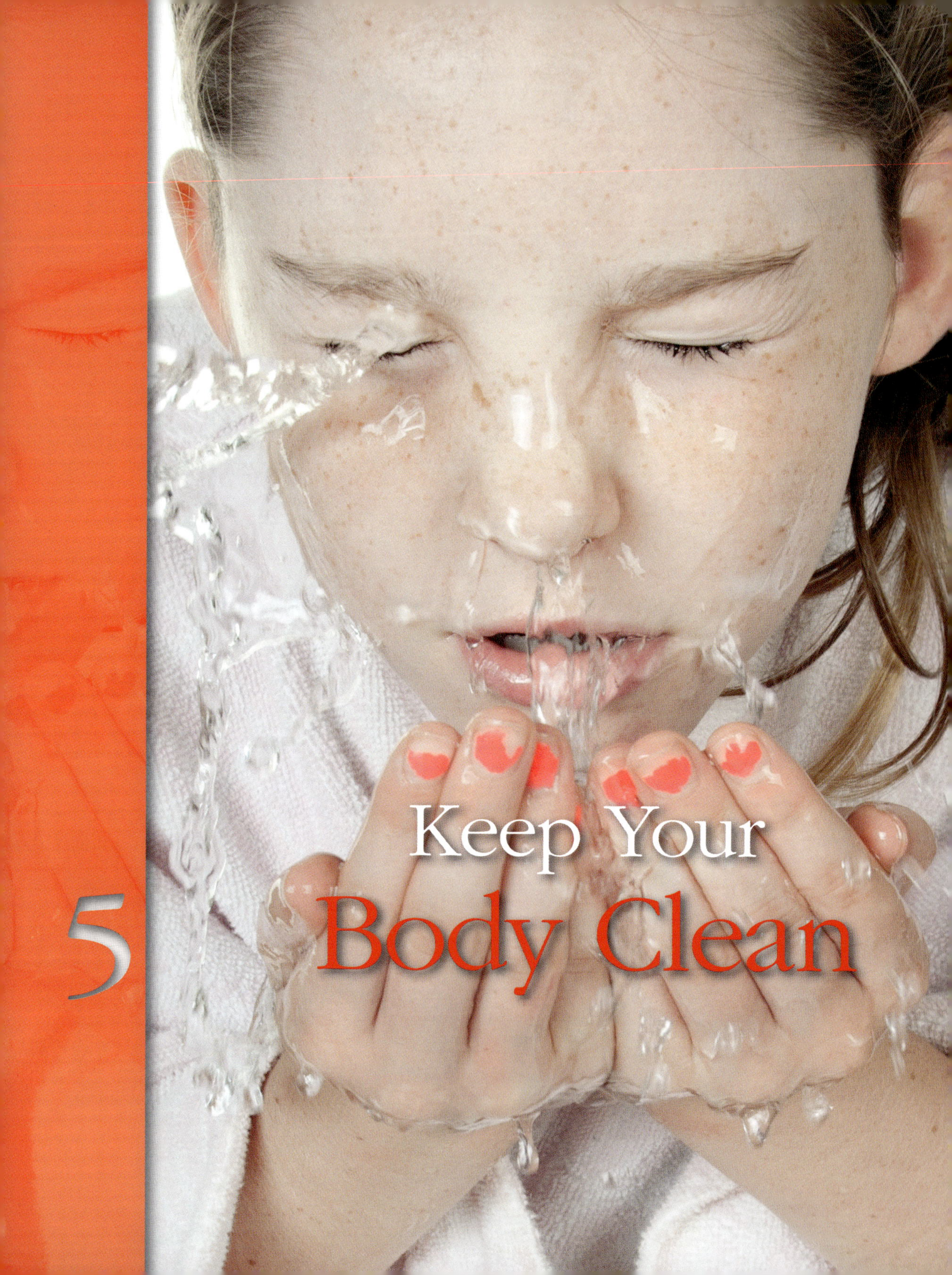

5 Keep Your Body Clean

Being clean isn't just about looking and smelling good. It helps keep you healthy.

Washing your hands, body, and hair with soap gets rid of germs. Brushing and flossing prevents your teeth from rotting.

Wash your hands with soap before you eat and after you use the toilet. Bathe or shower twice a week, or whenever you get dirty from playing. Brush your teeth after you wake up and before going to bed. Floss once a day.

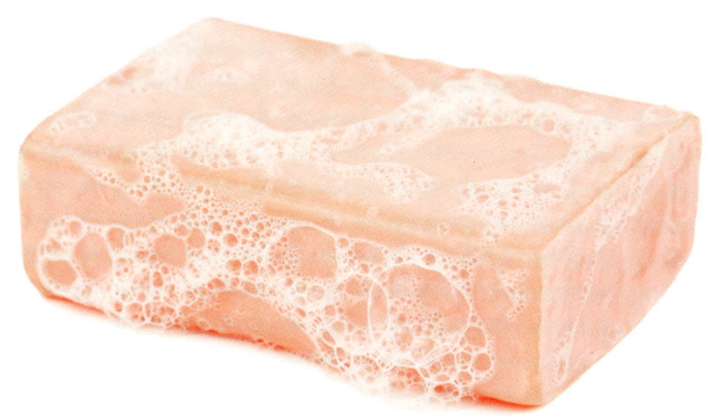

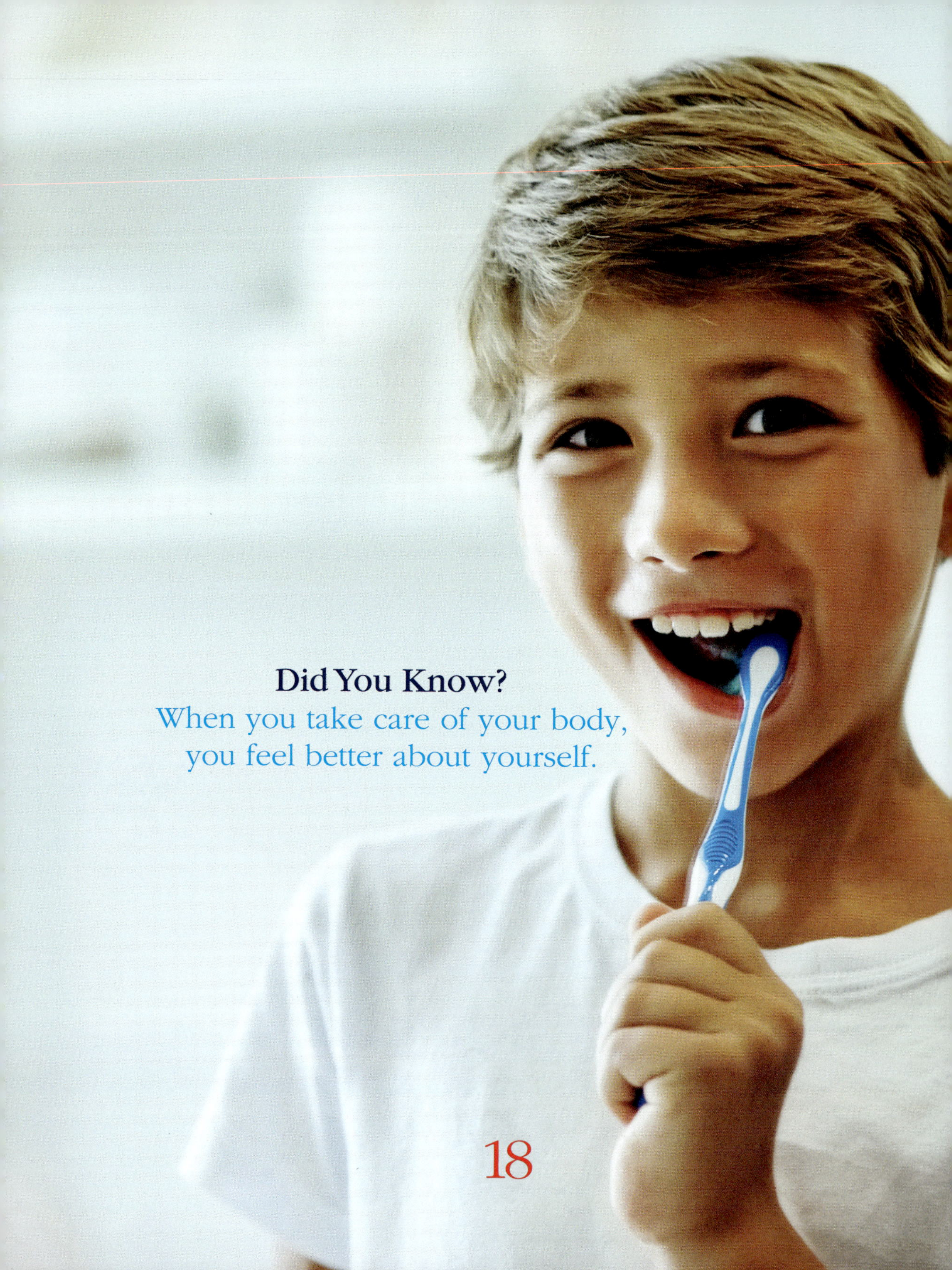

Did You Know?

When you take care of your body, you feel better about yourself.

Get Enough Sleep

6

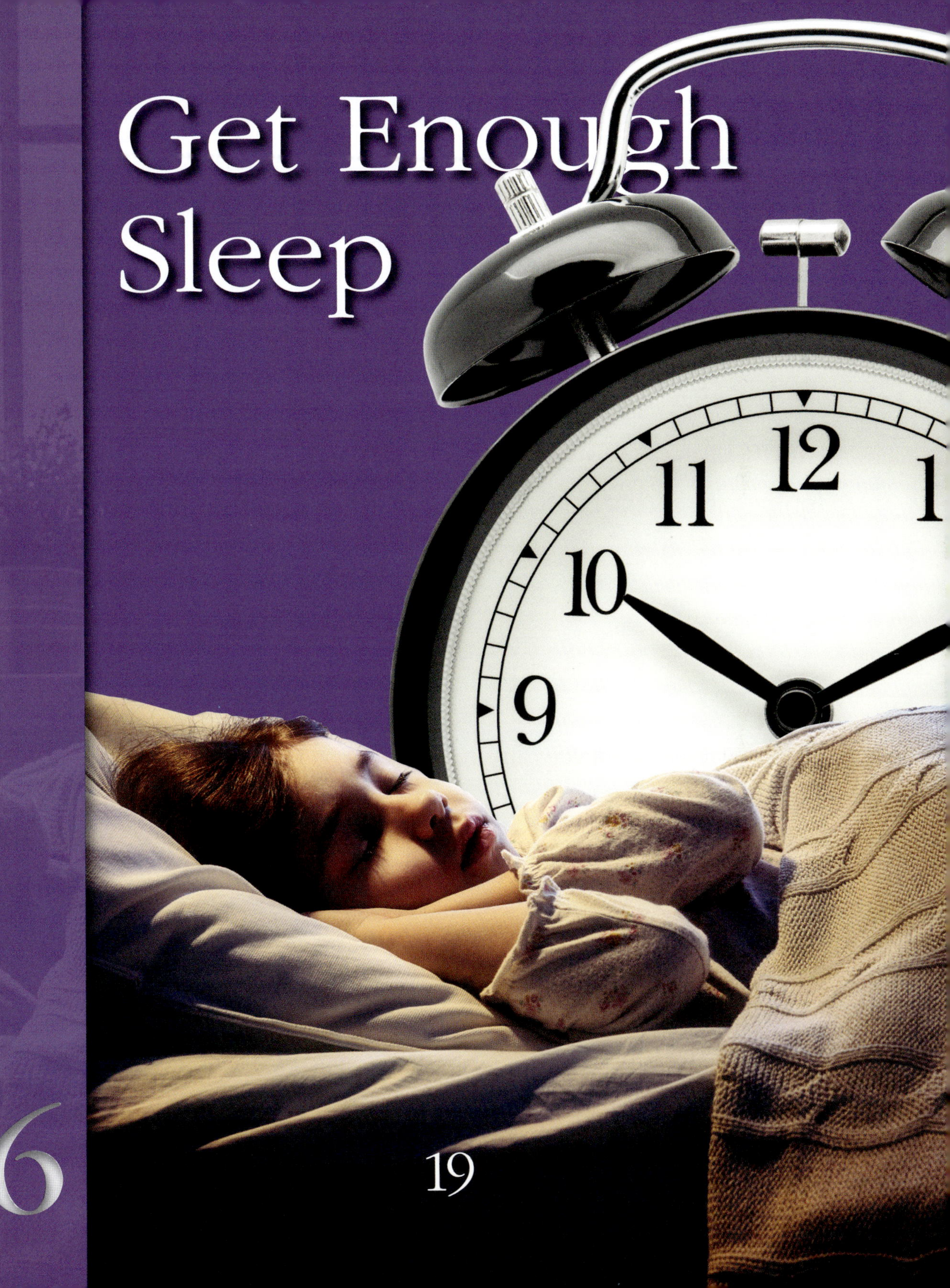

Kids your age need about 10 hours of sleep each night. Try to go to bed about the same time every day. Then your body will be used to falling asleep at that time.

When you get enough sleep, you're happier. You're more alert in school. You're less likely to get sick.

If you have trouble falling asleep, listen to soothing music or read a book. Being active during the day can help as well. Exercise wears out your body and mind.

Did You Know?
The blue light from screens and tablets can keep you from falling asleep. Avoid screens for at least an hour before bedtime.

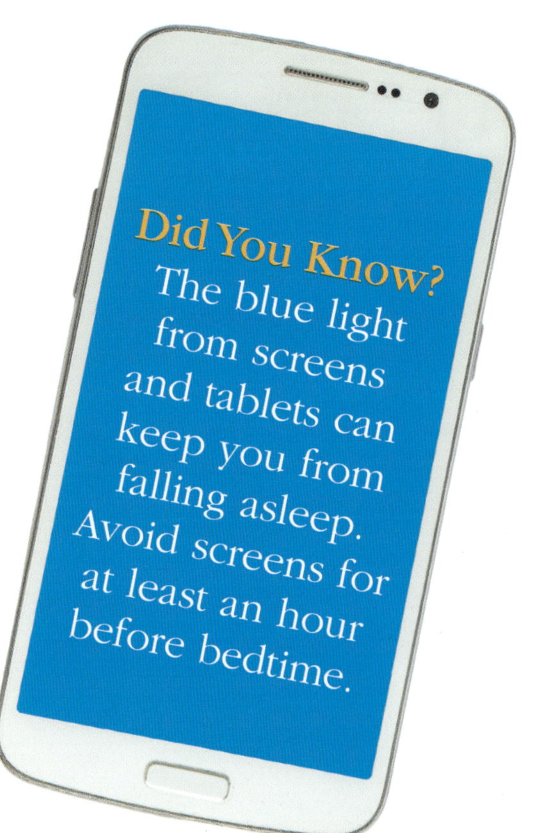

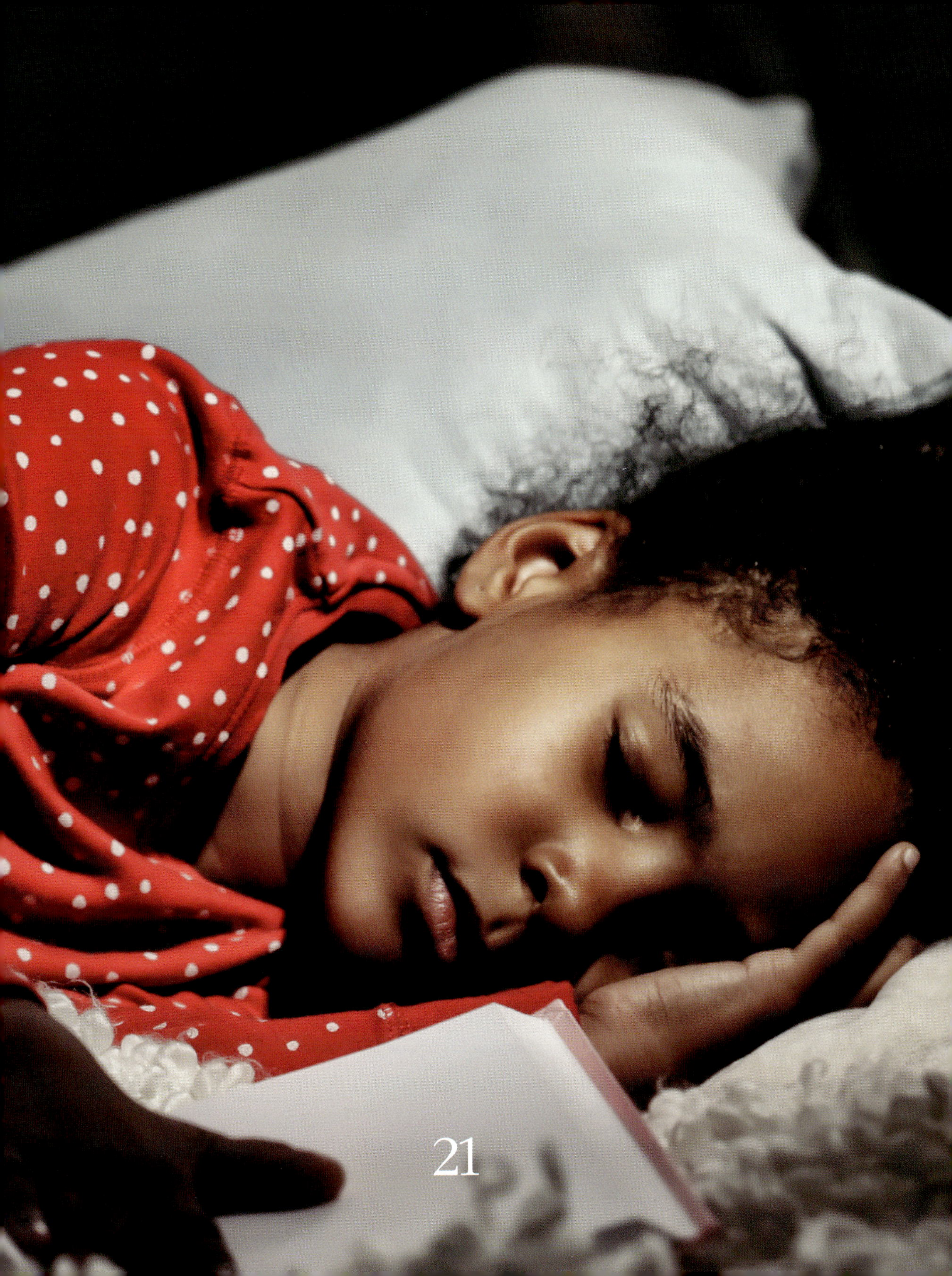

MORE TO EXPLORE

FANTASTIC FACTS

Being active gives you more energy, even when you're tired.

Drinking water can improve your mood and energy.

Walking outdoors can boost your self-esteem.

Yoga can improve your thinking abilities.

Reading before bed can be relaxing and help you fall asleep faster.

Laughing increases blood flow. This is good for your heart.

MORE TO EXPLORE

COOL COMPARISONS

How much sleep do people need?

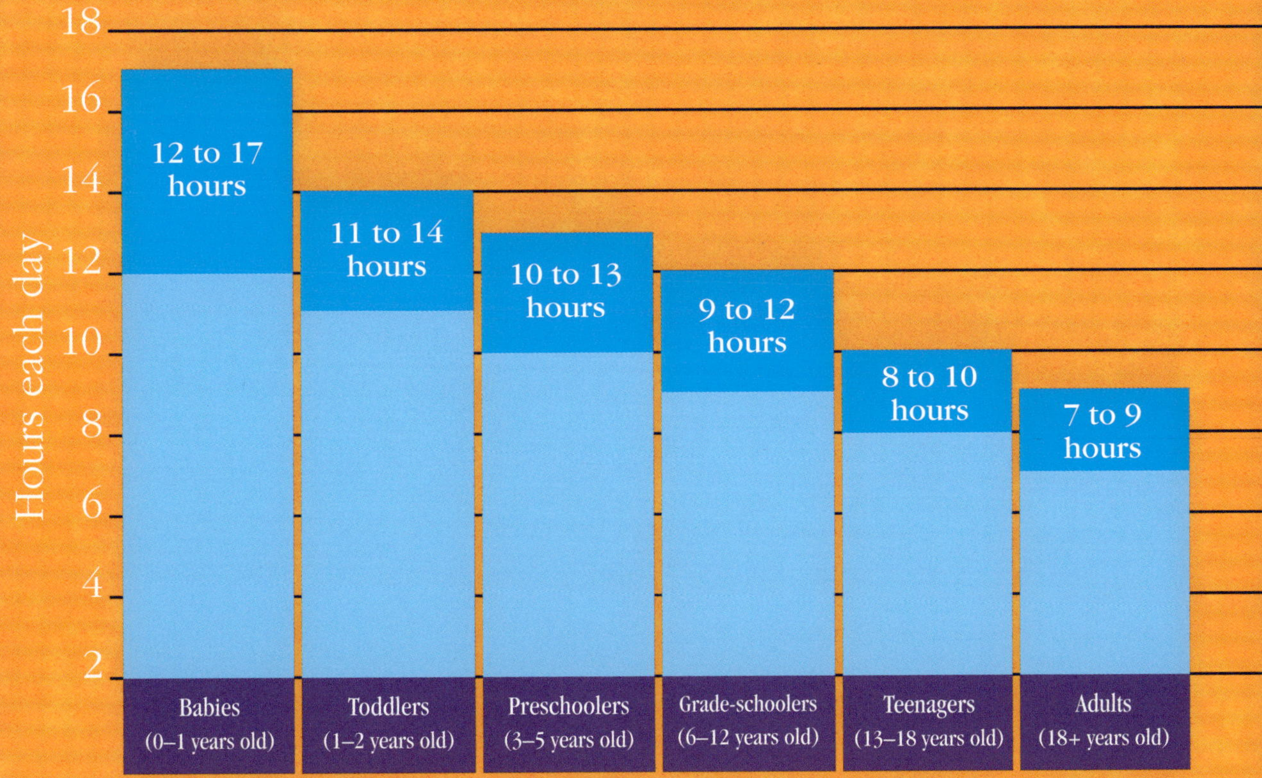

MORE TO EXPLORE

RESOURCES

Glossary

alert (uh-LURT) Able to think clearly and notice things.

habit (HAB-it) Something that you do often in a regular and repeated way.

immune system (i-MYOON SISS-tuhm) The system in your body that protects you from infections and diseases.

meditation (med-i-TAY-shuhn) To spend time in quiet thinking.

nutrient (NOO-tree-uhnt) A substance in food that is needed to be healthy.

self-esteem (SELF ess-TEEM) The feeling of respect for yourself.

strategy (STRAT-uh-jee) Thinking ahead with careful planning.

tension (TEN-shun) A nervous or anxious feeling.

Read More

Audra, Janari. *Physical Health in Our World.* New York: PowerKids Press, 2022.

Brundle, Harriet. *Sleep: Why We Rest and Recharge to Refuel.* Minneapolis: Bearport Publishing Company, 2021.

Index

being active, 5, 11, 20, 22
cleanliness, 17
food, 11
friends, 8
immune system, 8
relaxing, 14
self-esteem, 8, 18, 22
sleeping, 14, 20, 23
water, 12, 22

TOP RANK is published by Black Rabbit Books, P.O. Box 227, Mankato, MN, 56002.

• Top Rank is an imprint of Black Rabbit Books. • Edited by Alissa Thielges • Designed by Danny Nanos • Photographs © Getty: Cheryl Casey, 16; Shutterstock: ANURAK PONGPATIMET, 15, Bianca Grueneberg, 5, Evgeny Bakharev, 13, fizkes, 14, Focus no.5, 20, HordynskiPhotography, 12, Monkey Business Images, 2–3, 9, monticello, 11, Oleksandr Lysenko, cover, Patrick Foto, 6–7, Pavel K, 8, PeopleImages.com – Yuri, A 18, Pixel-Shot, 21, Prostock-studio, 8, 10, Sergey Novikov, 4, stable, 19, Valentina Razumova, cover, Vova Shevchuk, 17, Yuganov Konstantin, 19 • Printed in the United States of America

Library of Congress Cataloging-in-Publication Data: Names: Snow, Peggy, author. | Title: Healthy habits / by Peggy Snow. | Description: Mankato, MN: Black Rabbit Books, [2025] | Series: Top rank: healthy and happy | Ages 8–11 | Grades 4–6 | Identifiers: LCCN 2023058216 | ISBN 9781632357984 (library binding) | ISBN 9781645820765 (ebook) | Subjects: LCSH: Health behavior in children—Juvenile literature. | Classification: LCC RJ47.53 .S59 2025 | DDC 613/.0432—dc23/eng/20240125 | LC record available at https://lccn.loc.gov/2023058216